Brain Sharp

100 Exercises To Build A Better Brain And Keep Your Brain Sharp At Any Age

SAI RUDRA

ISBN: 9798710530917

TABLE OF CONTENT

INTRODUCTION

It's not all about heart health, healthy eating, blood pressure and BMI checks, and consistent workouts — all the healthy lifestyle practices that are excessively drilled into our brains. We need to take a moment to think about the brain itself; which is the control unit of our body's activities and the root of human intelligence.

This is because as people age, their thinking skills decline. They lose their cognitive abilities and tend to become more forgetful. What then is the use of staying fit and trim at the age of 70, when your memory and alertness is under a strain?

Your brain works hard. It uses about 25% of your body's energy. It needs to be exercised. When you exercise your brain, you are forming good memory habits. There's no better time to begin this. Just as you wouldn't wait until your muscles are flabby to begin to work them; or until your blood pressure go through the roof to begin exercises and healthy dieting, it is good practice to build a sharp brain right now and keep it sharp.

There are benefits to a quick start: it will help you perform better at your job or at school, and improve your memory and overall brain health in the future. Your brain will then be equipped to handle the inevitable deterioration that age brings without straining your memory.

Brain exercises strengthen your mind, which in turn boosts your memory and thinking skills. It reduces stress, improves your self-confidence, and makes you smarter and more independent; not to mention the tremendous benefit of maintaining your cognitive abilities as you age.

The exercises in this book are varied; and deliberately so to ensure that your brain is well-exercised and kept sharp. There are exercises to stimulate creative thinking, logical thinking, lateral thinking, memory and problem-solving; and they appear in form of practical puzzles, crypomath problems, memorization games, and grand riddles.

There are brain-racking exercises that will make you think and think to come up with a solution. There are also the easy and not-so easy exercises. There's something for everyone in here. So get ready to squeeze your minds, solve problems and express views and feelings appropriately.

Have fun!

Brain Sharp Exercises

1.

You are a competitor in a linear race. You run and then overtake the last runner. In which position are you now?

(a) Last

(b) Third to last

(c) Second to last

(d) Cannot say since the number of runners is not Known

(e) Cannot be determined because this is an ambiguous Question

2.

How much dirt is there in a hole 4 feet deep, 61/2 feet long, and 3 feet wide?

3.

A man buys a new car and hurries home to tell his wife. He goes the wrong way up a one-way street, almost runs into 6 people, goes onto the sidewalk, and takes a shortcut through a park. A policeman sees all his movements and still doesn't arrest him. Why didn't he?

4.

Can you solve this in a few seconds?

Which is greater, 3/7 or 7/16?

5.

Tongue Twisters

Improve your memory by saying these tongue twisters:

Freshly-fried flying fish.

Which wristwatches are Swiss wristwatches?

Many an anemone sees an enemy anemone.

Unique New York.

6

What is full of holes, but still holds lots of water?

7.

If I am holding a bee, what do I have in my eye?

8.

Read these aloud to uncover the cryptic meaning. YY = two Ys

YY UR

YY UB

I C U R

YY 4 ME

9.

The Big Accident

At the bottom of a large hill more than 50 cars were involved in a large accident. Some cars were overturned, while others were left to rest on top the other cars. It was such a large pile-up that even a couple of military vehicles as well as a fire truck ended up being involved in the crash. What caused the big wreck?

10.

How many books can enter into an empty backpack?

11.

What is the next letter in the following series: s t n o j k g h?

(a) c

(b) g

(c) d

(d) e

(e) f

12.

Put these statements in the right order:

(a) A woman tries on a dress.

(b) A woman buys a hat.

(c) A man buys a dress.

(d) A woman returns a dress to a store.

(e) A man gives his wife a present.

13.

Writing a Little a Lot

A man sits down on his big chair every two weeks and writes two words on 60 sheets paper. Why does he do this?

14.

An explorer found a silver coin marked 7 BC. On getting it examined, he discovered it was a forgery. Why?

15.

A doctor's son's father was not a doctor. How come?

16.

Everyone working at a carwash works at the same speed. Eight people can wash 50 cars in 60 hours. How many hours can four people wash 100 cars?

(a) 30

(b) 60

(c) 120

(d) 240

(e) 360

17.

A little boy kicks a soccer ball. It goes 9 feet and still comes back to him. How is this possible

18.

Ryan has some very silly dreams. On a certain night, he dreamt that he was a clown and when he awoke, his nose was a little red. Another night, he dreamt he was a king, only to discover when he was up that he was wearing his quilt like a robe. Tonight, he dreamt he was sleepwalking! What next?

19.

If a five-cent coin and a ten-cent coin is thrown into the air and one of them lands as a head, what's the probability that the five-cent coin will land as a head?

(a) 1/3

(b) 1/2

(c) 2/3

(d) 3/4

(e) 7/8

20.

A deaf beggar had a brother who died. What relation was the deaf beggar to the brother who died? Do not say "Brother", because it's *definitely* not the answer!

21.

Think Out Of The Box

Can you find out what is missing?

1 3 5

2 4 ?

Hint: It's not six. Think out of the box.

22.

Walking down a road, you come to a fork. One path leads to death; the other path to eternal happiness. You don't know which is which. At the centre of the fork, you see two brothers who know which road leads to which. One brother always tells the truth and the other always lies. You can only ask them one question. How would you determine which road to take?

23.

A man dressed in all black walks down a country lane. Suddenly, a large black car without its lights on comes round the bend and screeches to a stop. How did the car know he was there?

24.

A man drove all the way from San Francisco to New York. At the end of the trip he discovered he had a flat tire from the very start of his journey. Yet his car was totally unaffected by it? How is this possible?

25.

I am used to bat with, despite that, I never get a hit. I'm near a ball, but it is never thrown. What am I?

26.

X is the father of Y. But Y is not the son of X. Explain.

27.

It takes Sean 4 hours to do a job. It takes Peter 2 hours to do the same job. How many such jobs could they do together in 4 hours?

28.

Make "one word" from all the jumbled letters below:

o r e n o d w

29.

The Burglar

A man was wanted for burglarizing several businesses. Surveillance footage from the businesses showed this man's face clearly and the local TV Station repeatedly showed this footage to viewers. There were even "wanted" posters around the vicinity which were posted by the local police department to help catch the burglar. However, when the man was spotted by two police officers familiar with the burglaries, he was not arrested. What happened?

30.

What's wrong with this advertisement: "Shop early and avoid the crowds?"

31.

What day follows the day before yesterday if two days from now will be Sunday?

32.

A plumber, a hat maker and a lawyer were walking down the street. Who had the biggest hat?

33.

What's special about July 6, 1989, specifically at 23:45 PM?

34.

Mystery Weight Loss (lateral thinking)

A man enters a room and presses a button. Within seconds he instantly loses 20 pounds. How did he lose the weight?

35.

Why Are Manhole Covers Round And Not Square?

36.

What is the next number in the following sequence?

0 0 1 2 2 4 3 6 4 8 5?

(a) 12

(b) 8

(c) 10

(a) 6

(e) 14

37.

What gets wetter & wetter the more it dries?

38.

Logical Clock Problem

Palindrome is when something reads the same forwards or forward. Now a digital clock's time is palindromic (like 12:12). What's the minimum interval between 2 times that are palindromic?

39.

Find a word that has the same meaning when a prefix is placed before the word.

40.

A man opened the door, screamed, and then was found dead minutes later. However there were no gunshots heard in the area. What happened?

41.

Logic Thinking Puzzle

Mr. Red, Mr. Blue, and Mr. White meet at a restaurant for lunch. They are wearing different color of shirts under their coats (red, blue, or white shirt). Mr. Blue says, 'Hey, we are all wearing different colored shirts from our names, did you all notice that?' The man wearing the white shirt looks around and says, 'Wow, Mr. Blue, that's right!'

Can you tell who is wearing what color shirt?

42.

How can a man go eight days without sleep?

43.

Out of 3 females and 3 males, 3 people at random enter an empty room. What is the probability that there are two males and one female in the room now?

44.

Insert the mathematical symbols +, -, × and ÷) in between the numbers to get the accurate result? How can you do this?

2 4 6 8 = 20

2 4 6 8 = 28

2 4 6 8 = 6

45.

What am I if I only lie down once – when I die?

46.

Riddle: How many letters are in the alphabet?

47.

If you are running a race, and you pass the person in second, what place are you in?

48

Rearrange these statements accordingly:

(a) The ship stopped to anchor in Commander Bay.

(b) A boy awoke and saw a sea lion.

(c) A boy went ashore and napped in a meadow.

(d) A boy did not tell what he had seen.

(e) A boy got a job on a ship.

49.

A farmer has 19 sheep and all but 9 die. How many are left?

50.

How far can you walk into the woods?

51.

If I have 3 dimes, 3 nickels and 3 quarters, how many ways can I make change for $1.00?

(a) 3

(b) 2

(c) 1

(d) 4

(e) 5

52.

A girl has just enough money to buy 3 sweaters and 2 skirts, or 3 skirts and no sweaters. The sweaters are the same price, and all skirts are the same price. What is the maximum number of sweaters she can buy if she buys only one skirt?

53.

Can a man legally marry his widow's sister in the state of Mississippi?

54.

What word of five letters has only one left when two letters are removed?

55.

What English word has three consecutive double letters?

56.

You see a boat filled with people. You take a second look, but this time around you don't see a single person on the boat. Why?

57.

CryptoMath II

Work out the numbers each asterisk represents. The numbers used are 1 through 9 only, and no number is used twice (not even the answer).

* *__* = **, then minus** = 16

58.

Walk on the living, they don't even mumble. But walk on the dead, they mutter and grumble. What are they?

59.

Why couldn't Mozart find his teacher?

60.

How do you fit 10 horses into 9 stalls

61.

What can you infer from this sentence? "Since every child I know likes ice cream, M must also like ice cream."

(a) M likes anything sweet.

(b) M is a child.

(c) The speaker doesn't know many children.

(d) The speaker saw M eat ice cream

(e) The speaker is a good friend of M's.

62.

It's shorter than the rest, but when you're happy, you raise it up like it's the best. What is it?

63.

Logical Thinking Riddle

I have 100 coins in my purse.

What is the least number of coin(s), expected in order to ensure each coin touched exactly three other coins.

64.

Name three words that end in "DOUS."

65.

People buy me to eat, but never eat me?

66.

Proverb: Don't _____________ horses while crossing a

_____________.

67.

If you had only one match, and entered a dark room containing an oil lamp, a candle, some newspapers, and a wood stove, which would you light first?

68.

A barrel of water weighs 20 pounds. What must you add to it to make it weigh 12 pounds?

69.

When can you add two to eleven and get one as the answer?

70.

A doctor's son's father was not a doctor. How is this possible?

71.

What always ends everything?

72.

South African Proverb: If you are looking for a fly in your food it means that you are ______________.

73.

On your grandpa's desk is a 12-hour digital clock. The number for the hour reads the same as the number for the minute, all the time. Example 6:06 7:07, 10:10. What is the time difference between such times?

(a) 101 minutes

(b) 61 minutes

(c) 60 minutes

(d) 49 minutes

(e) 11 minutes

74.

Which of these two sentences is correct: "The yolk of the egg is white" or "the yolk of the egg are white?"

75.

Very few people keep me as straight as can be. Most of the time, I am curved or slightly bent. Your sadness causes me to bend further, usually, but don't bend me for long, as I may never be able to straighten out again fully. What am I?

76.

In the sentence below, count the number of times the letter F appears.

"Finished files are the result of years of scientific research combined with the experience of years."

77.

A murderer is sentenced to death. There are three rooms he must choose from: the first is a room full of raging fires; the second has assassins waiting with loaded weapons; and the third gas lions who haven't eaten in years. Which room is the safest?

78.

Take 1,000. Add 40. Add another 1,000. Add 30. Add 1,000 again. Add 20. Add 1,000. And add 10. What is the total?

(a) 4,900

(b) 5,000

(c) 4,100

(d) 4,000

(e) None of the above 79.

There are five cattle head in a paddock. A rancher comes into the paddock and goes out with two heads. How many are left in the paddock

80.

What is the next number in the series?

9, 15, 23, 33, ?

81.

Vietnam proverb: If you want to gather a lot of knowledge, act as if you are ___________________.

82.

You have 20 blue socks and 20 red socks in your drawer. You reach into the drawer without looking at the socks, what is the minimum amount of socks you must take out to ensure that you have a pair of socks of the same color?

(a) 4

(b) 3

(c) 1

(d) 41

(e) 10

83.

How are a jeweler and a jailer alike?

84.

Proverb: The frog does not ______________ the pond
in which he ____________.

85.

A woman's two sons were born on the same hour of
the same day and of the same year. However, they
weren't twins. How can you explain this.

86.

What flowers can be found between the nose and the
chin?

87.

Peter Ollie was asked how old he was. "In two years
I'll be twice as old as I was six years ago." How old is
Peter?

88.

What is the best exercise for losing weight?

89.

Proverb: From _____________ beginnings come great _____________.

90.

Liar Truth Riddle

Simon is a strange liar.

He lies on six days of the week, but on the seventh day he always tells the truth.

These are the statements he made on three successive days:

Day 1: "I lie on Monday and Tuesday."

Day 2: "Today, it's Thursday, Saturday, or Sunday."

Day 3: "I lie on Wednesday and Friday."

On which day does Simon tell the truth?

91.

French Proverb: With enough "ifs" we could put Paris into a ___________.

92.

What ancient invention still used in parts of the world today enables people to see through walls?

93.

Which is better: "The house burned down" or "The house burned up"?

94.

What's black when you get it, red when you use it, and white when you're all through with it?

95.

What's the answer when you divide 40 by 1/2 and add 20?

96.

A boy and a doctor went fishing. The boy was the doctor's son, but the doctor wasn't the boy's father. Who is the doctor?

97.

A certain orchestra has exactly three times as many string musicians as musicians who are playing wind instruments. Go through the following and figure out the combined number of string and wind musicians in this orchestra.

(a) 27

(b) 28

(c) 29

(d) 30

(e) 31

98.

It is mid-night and Mr. Jones is fast asleep in his hotel room. The telephone beside his bed rang. He wakes up, picks up the phone, and said "Hello." He puts the phone down beside him and goes back to sleep. Who had telephoned him?

99.

Logic Puzzle

A dead body is found outside a multistory company. The case is reported and a homicide detective is called on the crime scene.

He looks at the body and then towards the building. The body is positioned in a way that makes it evident that the victim committed suicide. The detective goes to the first floor of the building and then walks in the direction of the dead body, opens the window and toss a coin in the air.

He goes to second floor and again repeats the process. He continues to do this until he is done on all the floors. Afterwards, he returns back to the floor and tells his team that it is a murder.

How did he deduce that?

100

A sheep pen contains a bunch of sheep. Some of them are ewes. The number of sheep heads multiplied by the number of sheep hooves multiplied by the number of ewes' tongues equals 200. How many sheep are there, and how many of them are ewes?

ANSWERS & EXPLANATIONS

Answer 1

(e) You can't overtake someone who is last

Answer 2

None—otherwise it wouldn't be a hole.

Answer 3

The man was walking

Answer 4

7/16 is greater.

Multiply 16 × 3 and 7 × 7 in the fractions. 48 < 49 so

3/7 < 7/16

Answer 6

A sponge.

Answer 7

Beauty (from the proverb, "Beauty is in the eye of the beholder.)

Answer 8

YY UR - too wise you are

YY UB - two wise you be

I C U R - I see you are

YY 4 ME - too wise for me

Answer 9

The cars, the trucks, and other vehicles involved in the accident are simply toys in the midst of a child's playtime.

Answer 10

Just one; then the backpack isn't empty

Answer 11

(d) e

The sequence is arranged in pairs: st no jk gh

There's a pattern: gh (i) jk (lm) no (pqr) st

The letters in parentheses goes up by one letter in the sequence.

This way, the next two letters in the original sequence must be e, f, since the pattern will be preserved: ef (no letters) gh (i) jk (lm) no (pqr) st

Answer 12

c, e, a, d, b

Answer 13

The man is a small business owner with 60 employees on his payroll. Every fortnight, he signs name on their payroll checks.

Answer 14

The label BC only could have come into usage after 0 BC.

Answer 15

The doctor is the son's mother.

Answer 16

(d) 240

Explanation: If 8 people can wash 50 cars in 60 hours, this means 4 people can wash 50 cars in 120 hours. It would take twice as much time to wash, since there are half as many people to wash. Thus, it would take four people 240 hours, twice as long, to wash 100 cars, since there are twice as many cars now.

Answer 17

He kicked it straight up into the air

Answer 18

When he woke up he was in the yard!

Answer 19

(c) 2/3

Explanation: Probability is the favorable number of possible outcomes divided by the total number of possible outcomes.

Now one of the coins lands as a head, so the total number of ways this is possible is:

Five-cent head, ten-cent head

Five-cent head, ten-cent tail

Five-cent tail, ten-cent head

We cannot get a possibility of a ten-cent tail and ten-cent tail mix since one of the coins must be a head.

This leaves us with three possibilities.

Next is to find the favorable ways the five-cent coin will land as a head and this are:

Five-cent head, ten-cent head

Five-cent head, ten-cent tail

That is two ways out of three possible ways. The probability is c, which is 2/3.

Answer 20

The deaf beggar was the sister of her brother, who died.

Answer 21

"R", which stands for reverse, from the gear stick of your car! Pay attention next time!

Answer 22

If the path on the right leads to eternal happiness, for instance. Both brothers when asked will tell you the exact same thing: "the left path leads to eternal happiness."

What to do? Simply pick the opposite of what they both say. This is because one is telling the truth about it being a lie, and one is lying about it being the truth."

Answer 23

It was day time.

Answer 24

It was his spare tire that was flat.

Answer 25

Eyelashes.

Answer 26

Y is the daughter of X

Answer 27

3. In 4 hours Sean can do one job, and in 4 hours Peter can do two jobs.

Answer 28

One word

Answer 29

The man was in jail currently and the two police officers came to him to get a statement for his impending trial.

Answer 30

There aren't usually crowds in the early hours.

Answer 31

Thursday

 "Now" must be Friday, since two days from Friday is Sunday.

So in the phrase "the day before yesterday."
Yesterday is Thursday since now (today) is Friday.
"The day before yesterday "is Wednesday, and the

"day that follows the day before yesterday" is Thursday.

Answer 32

The one with the biggest head.

Answer 33

It could be written as 23:45 6/7/89 or 23456789

Answer 34

The room the man enters is an elevator. He presses the button and the elevator starts to accelerate downward. This acceleration changes his apparent weight temporarily, making it possible for him to lose 20 pounds in seconds.

Answer 35

Manhole covers are round to ensure they don't fall into the manholes. Square covers manholes if held diagonally, could be dropped into the manhole.

Answer 36

(c) 10

These are two alternating sequences: 0, 1, 2, 3, 4, 5 and 0, 2, 4, 6, 8.

Answer 37

A towel.

Answer 38

2 minutes (between 9:59 and 10:01)

Answer 39

PASSIVE

Answer 40

The man was on an airplane. He opened the door and he fell to his death.

Answer 41

Blue could only be wearing white or red. Since we know someone else is wearing the white shirt, it follows that Mr. Blue could only be wearing the red shirt.

Mr. White could have only been wearing a blue or a red shirt, and red is already taken, so Mr. White is wearing a blue shirt.

Mr. Red now has to be wearing a white shirt.

Answer 42
By sleeping during the night time

Answer 43
9/20

Answer 44
$2 + 4 + 6 + 8 = 20$

$2 + 4 \times 6 - 8 = 28$

$2 \times 4 \times 6 \div 8 = 6$

Answer 45
A tree

Answer 46
11 (t-h-e a-l-p-h-a-b-e-t).

Answer 47

Second place.

Answer 48

e, a, c, b, d

Answer 49

9. Remember it states: "all but 9 die."

Answer 50

Halfway—after that, you're walking out of the woods.

Answer 51

(b) 2

Answer 52

Six 3Sw + 2Sk = 3Sk. So, 3Sw = 1Sk.

Answer 53

No, because he's dead.

Answer 54

Stone.

Answer 55

Bookkeeper.

Answer 56

The boat has not sunk. All the people on the boat are married.

Answer 57

57 - 9 = 48, then minus 32 = 16

Answer 58

Leaves.

Answer 59

Because the teacher was Hayden.

(Hayden, Hiding)

Answer 60

[t] [e] [n] [h] [o] [r] [s] [e] [s]

Answer 61

(b) M is a child

Answer 62

A thumb.

Answer 63

4

3 placed flat on the table in a triangle (touching each other) and put the fourth one on top of them in the middle.

Answer 64

Don't let your mind play tricks on you. It is DOUS not "doos". Therefore answers are: stupendous, tremendous, or horrendous.

Answer 65

Plate

Answer 66

Don't change horses while crossing a stream

Answer 67

The match.

Answer 68

Holes.

Answer 69

When you add two hours to eleven o'clock, you get one o'clock!

Answer 70

The doctor is the son's mother.

Answer 71

The letter G.

Answer 72

If you are looking for a fly in your food it means that you are full

Answer 73

(d) 49 minutes.

 You're wrong if you got 61 minutes, or 101 minutes. The times closest to one another is 12:12 and 1:01, and the difference is 49.

Answer 74

Neither—the egg yolk is yellow!

Answer 75

Your posture.

Answer 76

Most people will overlook the word "OF" because usually "f" sounds like "fox. "of", however, makes a "v" sound. Additionally, due to overuse," of" is generally considered as one unit, overlooking the second letter/ sound.

Answer 77

The poor lions died of starvation.

Answer 78

c) 4,100

1,000 + 40 + 1,000 + 30 + 1,000 + 20 + 1,000 + 10
= 4,100.

Answer 79

Four. The rancher left with one head of cattle and his own head on his shoulders.

Answer 80

The series increases by an increasing number each time—i. e., by 6, then 8,then 10, then 12.

Answer 81

If you want to gather a lot of knowledge, act as if you are ignorant.

Answer 82

(b) 3

Answer 83

The jeweler sells watches and the jailer watches cells.

Answer 84

The frog does not drink up the pond in which he lives.

Answer 85

They were two of a set of triplets.

Answer 86

Tulips – "Two lips."

Answer 87

Peter is 14

Answer 88

Pushing yourself away from the table.

Answer 89

From small beginnings come great things.

Tuesday

Explanation: Simon tells the truth on only a single day of the week. Let say the statement made on day 1 is untrue, what this means is that he tells the truth on Monday or Tuesday.

Again, let say the statement made on day 3 is untrue, this shows that he tells the truth on Wednesday or Friday. We know that Simon tells the truth on only one day, so these statements cannot both be untrue.

Now exactly one of these statements must be true, and the statement on day 2 must be untrue.

Let say the statement on day 1 is true. This means that the statement on day 3 must be untrue, and goes to show that Simon tells the truth on Wednesday or Friday.

Therefore, day 1 is a Wednesday or a Friday and then day 2 is a Thursday or a Saturday. Then again, this would imply that the statement on day 2 is true, but this cannot be. From this we can conclude that the statement on day 1 must be untrue.

This means that Simon told the truth on day 3 and that this day is a Monday or a Tuesday. So day 2 is a Sunday or a Monday. Because the statement on day 2 must be untrue, we can conclude that day 2 is a Monday.

So day 3 is a Tuesday. Therefore, the day on which Simon tells the truth is Tuesday.

Answer 91
With enough "ifs" we could put Paris into a bottle.

Answer 92
A window.

Answer 93
Neither! No basis for comparison; they're both bad!

Answer 94
Charcoal.

Answer 95

100

Don't be careless. Watch what you are dividing.
You're not dividing by 2, you are dividing by 1/2. So
you have to know your basic skills. Diving by 1/2 is
like multiplying by two. So the answer is $(40 \times 2) +$
$20 = 80 + 20 = 100$.

Answer 96

The boy's mother.

Answer 97

(b) 28

Using symbols, let $S = 3W$. $S + W =$ Number of
string and wind musicians. Thus, $3W + W = 4W$ is
the number of string and wind musicians. The only
choice where W is a whole number is where $4W = 28$
$(W = 7)$.

Answer 98

The person who called him was the man in the room
next door, and the reason the man telephoned him
was that Mr. Jones had been snoring and disturbing
the man. As soon as Mr. Jones said "Hello" the man

next door realized that he was awake and that was all
he wanted.

51

Answer 99

He was able to deduce that after noticing that all the
windows in the direction of the body on all the floors
were closed. If the man had committed suicide, one
window must have been left open.

Answer 100

Five sheep, two of which are ewes.

Concluded